SMOKING AND ALCOHOL

Habits That Are Killing Us

by

PAUL POWELL

TABLE OF CONTENTS

INTRODUCTION

C ombined, smoking and drinking kill around three million people annually in just the United States alone. The things that we are choosing to do are the leading causes of death in the United States, and yet we continue to take part in them.

On top of the almost half a million people who are dying annually from smoking related issues, 15 million are suffering from smoke-related illnesses, and one in ten 13 to 17-year old's that are alive right now are expected to die from smoke related illnesses.

Of those that are dying prematurely of alcohol-related issues, 71 percent of them are men, and over half of their causes of death are binge drinking.

There was a time not so distant in our history that we were told that drinking and smoking would not adversely affect our health, but things have changed, and now we know that those who take part in these activities are dying at least 10 years before those that do not, on average.

That makes many of us ask if that cigarette, cigar, or drink is actually worth 10 years of our lives. This book is going to discuss in depth about these habits that we have chosen to take part in and how they are not only killing us but how they are affecting our health. It is also going to teach you why it is so hard for those who have picked up these habits to quit, as well as what you can do to increase your chances of quitting.

Many people do not even attempt to quit smoking or drinking because they feel that the damage is already done, but we are going to finish this book up by looking at the effects that quitting can have on your health as well, as your quality of life.

Now that we know that these habits are causing more deaths than anything else, it is time for us to step up and not only understand but also break these habits that are killing us.

CHAPTER 1:

PUFFING YOUR WAY TO AN EARLY GRAVE

Tobacco is dangerous. No matter how you are smoking it, the tobacco is going to do the same damage. Many people think that by switching to a pipe, cigars, or even a hookah, they are reducing their chances of suffering from tobacco-related illnesses, but the truth is, as long as the tobacco is there, so is the chance of you developing a tobacco-related illness.

In about the 50's, smoking was looked at differently. It was considered elegant, it was cheap, and there were a lot of advertisements on television. After years of finding that people were suffering from smoking-related diseases, the television advertisements started to slow down, but it seems that it was far too late.

Those that were alive during the 50's had become addicted to smoking and seemed to have passed it on to the next generation. Studies show that children whose parents smoke are actually two times more likely than other children to begin smoking in their late teens.

Those same studies have found that when it comes to influences that cause 13 to 21-year old's to start smoking, parents or older siblings smoking ranked number 1.

So besides influencing your children or younger siblings to smoke, what is the constant puffing doing to your body? As dramatic as it may sound, that little smoking stick is a slow killer that is doing huge amounts of damage to your body.

When it comes to the damage that can be done to a person's body from smoking, most people think about the respiratory system, and while this is not the only system or part of the body that is damaged, I do want to begin here.

When you inhale the smoke of a cigarette, pipe, or cigar, you are inhaling toxic materials that will do huge amounts of damage to your lungs. Coughing is the natural way that the lungs clear themselves. However, this natural process does not clear out the toxins that are taken in when smoking.

Because these toxins are trapped in the lungs, those that smoke have an increased occurrence of the flu and colds, as well as respiratory infections, such as bronchitis.

Chronic bronchitis can occur, causing the lining of the bronchial tubes to become inflamed, causing wheezing and making it difficult to breathe. COPD can also develop as well as emphysema. When a person smokes long-term, it can lead to lung cancer.

When you stop smoking, you will find that you will begin suffering from more congestion, pain, and wheezing for a little while.

On top of all of this, smoking does not just affect how you are breathing, but how those around you are breathing as well. Children of parents who smoke have a higher chance of suffering from respiratory disorders such as asthma and tend to wheeze or cough more than children of parents that do not smoke.

Nicotine causes the blood vessels in the body to tighten, making it harder for blood to flow through the body. Smoking also causes a rise in blood pressure, as well as a higher risk of forming blood clots. It also increases your chance of having a heart attack, stroke, and heart disease.

For those who care about their looks, it is important for them to understand that smoking can be the cause of wrinkles, changes in the skin, discoloration of the skin and nails, as well as premature aging. Smoking can change the color of your teeth, and it makes you, as well as your breath, smell bad.

Smoking also affects the digestive system. Starting at the mouth, smoking can cause inflammation in the gums, the loss of teeth, decaying of teeth, and an increase of cancer in the mouth, throat, and even the esophagus.

Smoking makes it harder for men to get an erection, as well as making it harder for both women and men to achieve an orgasm. Women who smoke have a higher chance of developing cervical cancer and tend to experience menopause earlier in life. Tobacco can also make it more difficult to conceive, cause placenta problems, low birth weight, and a higher risk of miscarriages.

When a baby is exposed to second-hand smoke the chances of them suffering from SIDS increases; they will suffer from more ear infections and even asthma attacks.

CHAPTER 2:

HOW IS ALCOHOL AFFECTING YOUR HEALTH

W hen most people think about drinking, they do not think about how it affects their health. In fact, they do not think of it as an addiction or bad habit at all. The reason for this is that while smoking has become a bit taboo, drinking is still widely accepted.

However, when you drink, the alcohol is absorbed directly into your bloodstream, which allows it to affect every area of your body. This means that drinking can cause serious risks to your health.

Even the smallest amount of alcohol can have an effect on your body and your health. When you drink, the alcohol is absorbed directly into the blood leaving just a small amount to be found in the urine, as well as on the breath. The rest of the alcohol is pushed through the body in the bloodstream. Of course, we all know that if we drink too much, we will become drunk, but not only does that put us in harm's way, but it also causes immense damage to our bodies.

You will absorb alcohol more slowly if you eat as you are drinking. This is especially true if the food contains high amounts of fat. However, even eating a high fat meal will not stop you from getting drunk and it will not stop the effects of the alcohol on your body.

Drinking too much alcohol can cause damage to the pancreas, causing it to release toxins into the body. One of the most common causes of pancreatitis is alcohol consumption.

We all know that the liver breaks down the harmful substances in the body and that does include alcohol. When a person takes part in excessive drinking, it can lead to hepatitis, which can lead to jaundice.

When the liver is inflamed for long periods of time, scar tissue will develop, and this scar tissue destroys the liver. When the liver is unable to break down toxins, they remain in the body and this can be life-threatening.

Women tend to absorb alcohol much quicker than men, however, they also process it more slowly, which means that they are at higher risk for liver damage than men are.

On top of all of this, drinking can also increase your chances of developing liver cancer no matter if you are male or female.

One of the first ways that alcohol affects your body is through the nervous system. You begin to slur your words, maybe stumble, and can suffer from impulse control. Alcohol can cause long term effects to your brain, cause seizures, and even shrink the frontal lobe of your brain.

The damage that it causes to your nervous system can cause numbness in your extremities that will last for the rest of your life. It can cause paralysis of the eyes, irritation to the mouth and tongue, diarrhea, lower metabolism, internal bleeding, ulcers, and many different types of cancer.

While it may seem in today's society that drinking is acceptable, even that it is a rite of passage into adulthood, or that it is sophisticated, it does just as much damage to the body as smoking if not more. We all know the effects that drinking can have on a fetus, the same effects that are caused by smoking, but we have somehow forgotten that it can kill us or damage our bodies, causing us to suffer from long-term illnesses.

CHAPTER 3:

WHY ARE THESE HABITS SO HARD TO KICK

E very day, thousands of people decide that they are going to quit smoking or drinking. They tell themselves that this is the last pack, or that this is the last drink. They create amazing plans that on paper look great, but when it comes down to it, they are unable to quit.

These same people may try to stop drinking or smoking multiple times, finding that each time they try, they fail.

So why is it so hard? Let's first talk about why it is so hard for so many people to quit smoking. There are hundreds of people who lay the cigarettes down and never pick them up again, but for those that are unable to do so, there has to be an underlying reason.

Nicotine is the reason that most people find it difficult to quit smoking, and this is why there are so many smoking cessation products available today. These products are supposed to replace the nicotine that people are getting from cigarettes and allow the person to slowly reduce the amount of nicotine that they are using.

Many people find that this is a healthier option than smoking because they are not inhaling all of the chemicals that are in cigarettes into their lungs.

Nicotine has been proven to be just as addictive as cocaine or heroin, which means that the person becomes not only physically addicted but emotionally addicted to the drug as well. Because of this addiction, it makes it very difficult for many people to stay away from nicotine after they decide to quit smoking. One of the main causes of this is because most people who smoke, know someone that does smoke or live in a home with another smoker.

Imagine if a person who was addicted to cocaine was around other people using cocaine all of the time. The chances of them being able to stay clean would drop dramatically.

When it comes to smoking, it is not as if you can avoid places that allow smoking. You will pass people smoking while you are walking through the park, while you are on break at work, and literally everywhere else in your life.

On top of this, many people who smoke use it to relieve or deal with stress. This means that when they become stressed when trying to smoke, they are unable to handle the stress because they never really learned how to deal with it any other way.

Nicotine causes pleasant feelings in the body, just like any other drug, these feelings replace the unpleasant feelings that the smoker was feeling, which makes the smoker want to use nicotine again, the next time that they experience unpleasant feelings.

Just like with other drugs, when a person is using nicotine, the person's body becomes used to the nicotine, which means that they have to use more of it in order to feel the same way next time. This is why many people will go from smoking one or two cigarettes per day to one or two packs per day.

When a person tries to quit smoking, they have to deal with nicotine withdrawal symptoms. These symptoms include dizziness which can last up to two days after quitting, depression, anger, frustration, anxiety, irritability, inability to sleep, nightmares, problems concentrating, boredom, or not knowing what to do with their hands, increase in appetite, weight gain, headaches, coughing, tiredness, and much more.

It is because of these withdrawal symptoms that most people begin smoking again. It is also important for you to know that if you are on any type of prescription medication, the doctor who prescribed it should know that you are smoking. This means that when you stop smoking, it can cause your prescription medication to act differently. It is important for you to talk to your doctor to ensure that if any of your medications will be affected that the doses can be adjusted.

Drinking can be just as difficult to stop as smoking. When a person first starts drinking, it can be very easy for them to stop drinking. However, once they become addicted, it becomes much harder, because just like any other drug, alcohol affects every part of your life.

One of the main reasons that many people find that it is hard for them to quit drinking is that they do not recognize that a problem exists. Most people who are addicted to alcohol will have no problem admitting that they enjoy having a drink, but they are unable to see that it is causing a problem in their lives.

There are some that may know that their drinking is causing issues, but they find it very difficult to quit. This may be because they have tried to quit in the past and struggled with the symptoms that they had to face, or it may be that they simply do not know how to deal with life without having a few drinks.

Of course, there are also those who feel that all they have to do is put the bottle down and they will be fine. They do not think that they are addicted to alcohol because they have never had any experience with addiction before.

It is important for you to understand that even though the alcohol companies claim that you can drink safely, there is not a safe amount of alcohol when it comes to damaging your body. Even one drink a day can cause extreme damage and even lead to death.

Many people drink for the same reason that people smoke. It makes all of the negative feelings that they have go away, and they are filled with a warm and pleasant feeling. The alcohol has become a way for them to deal with their feelings without having to really deal with them.

There are also those who feel that they cannot be themselves unless they have a few drinks. They may struggle with social interactions or feel uninhibited when they are drinking.

Just like when you stop using any other drug, when you stop using alcohol, you will suffer from withdrawal symptoms, and this is one of the major reasons that so many people find it hard to quit.

Most people who drink become fearful of recovery because they have heard stories about how difficult it can be for them when they are trying to quit. Just like any other drug, your body will crave the alcohol when you decide to quit.

It is important for you to change the way that you think about quitting. Yes, chances are that you are going to have some unpleasant symptoms for a few days, however, that is nothing compared to the life that you can have if you stop drinking right now.

Those who want to quit drinking have to change the way that they spend time with their friends. You see, you might find that the only think that you have in common with your friends is that you drink at the same bar. You may find after you quit drinking that you don't like a lot about the people you have been spending time with. You have to be prepared to make changes in your life and give up those people that you only have drinking in common with.

You will have to find something else to do on Friday night instead of sitting at the bar. This may have become a habit for you, but quitting drinking is going to allow you to spend your time doing more important things. You are going to be able to find hobbies that you enjoy and friends that you really do have something in common with.

There are many reasons that people drink, some of them are to deal with things that have happened to them in their lives, and when they try to quit, they have to deal with these events. If you find that you are having a hard time quitting because you have to deal with the events of the past, it is important for you to seek professional help.

Make sure that you have someone to talk to about what has happened that has caused you to drink. It does not have to be a psychologist, however, having one is advisable. If all else fails, there are rehabilitation centers that you can check yourself into which will help you through the detoxification process.

CHAPTER 4:

WHAT YOU CAN DO TO INCREASE YOUR

CHANCES OF QUITTING

A nyone who has ever tried to stop smoking knows how difficult it can be. Even the smallest thing can be a trigger to make you crave a cigarette.

Chances are that if you have been smoking for any length of time, you have been told how it can affect your health, how you can save money if you quit, how it can lead to death, and how it can cause cancer, but the fact remains the same, quitting is hard.

Over 80 percent of smokers have tried to quit smoking. This tells me that the majority of people who smoke, know that it is unhealthy, and it is something that they do not want to do, but they feel that they have no control over.

1 in 10 smokers have tried to quit by using medications. Many of these have been approved by the FDA, but what most studies find is that most smokers simply do not understand how to use them properly to ensure that they are as effective as possible.

However, studies have also shown that many people will attempt to quit smoking by using methods that have not been approved by the USDA. For example, many people will switch to light cigarettes in an attempt to quit. This is one of the reasons that the word "Light" has been taken off of cigarette packs. Switching to a different cigarette is not going to reduce the amount of nicotine that you are inhaling.

There are also many other options that people will turn to, such as electronic cigarettes and hypnosis. It is very important for you to know that electronic cigarettes do just as much damage if not more to your lungs as cigarettes do.

If you choose to use nicotine gum to quit smoking, it is important for you to chew the gum slowly. Place the gum between your teeth in the back of your mouth and allow the outer coating to dissolve. After the outside has dissolved, you can begin chewing, but if you chew too quickly, your body will not be able to absorb the nicotine.

When it comes to the patches, many people have tried them, however they do not follow the directions on the package. Most patches will tell you not to lower your dosage for at least 10 weeks. However, some people think that they can reduce the dosage of the patch much earlier.

If you want to be successful at quitting smoking and are using a patch, it is important for you to understand that you should not reduce the dosage of the patch unless you have gone for 14 days without having any cravings.

Many people will take the patch off if they slip and have a cigarette. However, this is not necessary. If you smoke a cigarette, do not let it get to you, simply try again and continue trying until you no longer smoke.

You can also reduce the dosage of your patch if you feel that you are having side effects from the patch. There are also people who avoid the patch because it gives them very vivid nightmares, however, instead of not using the patch altogether, it is better for you to use the patch during the day and take it off at night. You may find that you will need a piece of nicotine gum in the morning because your patch has not been on you all night. However, this is fine and you will not have to worry about getting too much nicotine in your system because the nicotine in the patch will take a little while to enter your system.

One thing that causes many people to give up on the NRT's is because they are so expensive. It is true that these smoking cessations are expensive, however, this is a short-term expense, and you have to remember how much money you are going to save in the end.

For the first few days up till the first few weeks, you are going to sweat a lot. You will sweat when you are hot, as well as when you are freezing. While your body works to rid the toxins from it, you are not only going to sweat it out, small amounts will be found in your urine as well as in your breath, which means that your breath will smell like alcohol.

As you sweat the toxins out, it is going to cause an odor. This is not the same type of odor that you would normally smell when someone is sweating, and you will probably need a very strong deodorant, body spray, and lots of water.

The next thing that you are going to have to deal with is the dreams. For many drinkers, sleeping and passing out are basically the same thing, however, when they stop drinking, most will find that they will begin having nightmares. After not dreaming for a long period of time, this may be terrifying, and it can interrupt sleep dramatically.

Another thing that you may notice is that while it was very easy to fall asleep with all of the toxins in your body, now your mind is awake at bedtime. You may have racing thoughts when you are trying to go to sleep, but there is a way to get through this. Listening to sleeping hypnosis or relaxing music while you are trying to fall asleep will help, or you might find that reading a book helps your mind to relax.

You have to remember that your brain is not only more active than it is used to being, but it is also in panic mode. Something has changed and your brain nor your body understand why you are not giving it the substance that you have allowed it to become addicted to.

One of the most common dreams that those recovering from alcohol addiction suffer from is that the dream they fall off the wagon so to speak and begin drinking again. One thing that you can easily learn how to do is to remind yourself that you are asleep in the middle of your dreams. Simply knowing that you are going to dream this will allow you to realize that it is a dream and help you to take control of it.

Going to the bathroom is another problem that you are going to have to deal with. You see, you probably have been replacing a lot of your calories with alcohol. This means that once you stop drinking and start eating again, you are going to have to deal with diarrhea. In order to avoid this symptom and make your chances of success much higher, begin by adding food to your diet slowly. Start with one food that is high in fiber, for example, broccoli, and eat that whenever you feel extra hungry. You can also add some whole grain bread to your diet in order to harden up your stools.

It is important that you have support while you are quitting drinking because your short-term memory is not going to work that well. This means that you are going to forget a lot of small things, such as where you put your keys. On top of this, you will find that you are on edge and feel like murdering someone for even the smallest mistake. You absolutely must have someone to talk to about this. Writing in a journal is also a great help.

CHAPTER 5:

WHAT HAPPENS TO YOUR

BODY WHEN YOU QUIT

The wonderful thing about quitting smoking is that within the first hour, your body begins to repair itself. Within the first 20 minutes of quitting smoking, your blood pressure, as well as your heart rate, will begin to drop back to normal. You will also notice that the temperature of the hands and the feet begin to rise back to a normal temperature.

Within 8 hours, smokers breath disappears and carbon monoxide levels decrease in the body allowing oxygen levels to increase. Within the first 24 hours of quitting smoking, the chances of you having a heart attack decrease, and within the first 48 hours, the nerve endings and taste buds begin to regrow, which is why many people find that food tastes better and they are more sensitive to smells. It only takes three days for you to begin to breathe better.

As time continues on, as long as you do not pick up another cigarette, your body will continue to work to remove the toxins, and your health will eventually be that of a person who has never smoked.

After you have gone through alcohol withdrawals, your body is going to begin repairing itself as well. One of the first things that you will notice as your body becomes more used to eating solid food is that you will not be as hungry as you used to be, and your meals will become smaller. For most people, that means a dramatic change in weight.

While you might have problems sleeping in the beginning, when you quit smoking, you will find that eventually, you will begin sleeping more soundly and waking up with more energy than before. This means that you will have an improved mood, an increase in concentration, and higher mental performance.

You will have to be careful that you do not replace the addiction to alcohol for one of sugar. If you do crave sugar, it is okay for you to have a small bit of dark chocolate, which you will find makes you feel good just like the alcohol did. You will have to keep this under control, and if you do, chances are that you are going to lose the extra weight that you have put on while ingesting excessive amounts of alcohol.

Your risk of developing cancer is going to drop dramatically, however, you will have to keep an eye on your heart and liver. If there is any damage that has gone undetected, it could affect your health later in your life. However, it will affect it much less if you stop drinking right now.

CONCLUSION

Drinking and smoking are two habits that many people have that are killing them, and many of them do not even realize the damage that is being done. I hope that within this book you have begun to understand the damage that is being done and you have learned a few ways to help you stop.

With thousands of people trying to quit both drinking and smoking every single day, I feel that it is important for us to show support for each other. If you are trying to quit, please let those around you know, and if you know someone that is trying to quit, it is important that you are supportive of them.

In order to get more support, some people will join groups such as AA, and you should never feel ashamed for doing this. You should feel proud of yourself for making the changes in your life that you know need to be made so that you can live the life that you have always dreamed of.

As you work through this process, remind yourself every day why you are quitting, and once you begin saving money from stopping, reward yourself with something that you have wanted but have not had the money to purchase due to your addiction.